Dharmendra Kumar
Pramod Kumar Sharma

Capsule: Solid Oral Dosage Form

Dharmendra Kumar
Pramod Kumar Sharma

Capsule: Solid Oral Dosage Form

Drug Delivery System

LAP LAMBERT Academic Publishing

Cover image: www.ingimage.com

Publisher:
LAP LAMBERT Academic Publishing
is a trademark of
Dodo Books Indian Ocean Ltd. and OmniScriptum S.R.L publishing group

120 High Road, East Finchley, London, N2 9ED, United Kingdom
Str. Armeneasca 28/1, office 1, Chisinau MD-2012, Republic of Moldova, Europe
Managing Directors: Ieva Konstantinova, Victoria Ursu
info@omniscriptum.com

Printed at: see last page
ISBN: 978-620-8-44185-2

TABLE OF CONTENT

CAPSULE: SOLID ORAL DOSAGE FORM

CAPSULES, SOFT

INTRODUCTION

Soft gelatin capsules (Softgels) provide the option of giving a liquid oral dose form in a solid shape. The chosen dosage form for new chemical entities with poor bioavailability due to poor water solubility as well as for the life-cycle extension reformulation of commercial pharmaceuticals is the softgel due to its capacity to boost bioavailability. The basics of softgel formulation, production, and product development are covered in this chapter. Review of recent developments in this dosage form is also included, including non-gelatin-based Softgels, Softgels with modified or controlled release, and Softgels in chewable form.

BACKGROUND

In comparison to conventional dosage forms like tablets, hard-shell capsules, and liquids, soft gelatin capsules (also known as soft elastic gelatin capsules, Liqui-Gels, or Softgels) have certain significant advantages. However, there are only a few producers of Softgels worldwide because of technological, financial, and patent restrictions.

The major advantages of Softgels include the following:

- ❖ Bioavailability has been improved. More than 40% of newly discovered NCEs (new chemical entities) have good membrane permeability but poor aqueous solubility (i.e., Bio-pharmaceutics Classification System II). The solubility and thus bioavailability of the compound may be improved by formulating the NCE in solution inside a Softgel (e.g., lipid-based) or in micro/nano emulsion.
- ❖ Improve drug stability (protection against oxidation, photo degradation, and hydrolysis in lipophilic systems).

- ❖ Patient compliance/customer preference, as well as pharmaceutical elegance According to the findings of studies conducted over the years, consumers prefer Softgels for their ease of swallowing, perceived speed of delivery, lack of unpleasant odor or taste, and modern appearance.
- ❖ Outstanding dose uniformity.
- ❖ Improved tamper evidence (tampering leads to puncturing and visible leakage).
- ❖ Product differentiation through safer handling of highly potent or cytotoxic drug compounds (through selection of novel shapes, colours, and sizes).
- ❖ Outstanding product life-cycle management. For instance, product enhancement through faster onset of action.
- ❖ Softgels, on the other hand, have few disadvantages. These are some examples:Specialized manufacturing equipment requirements.
- ❖ Higher manufacturing cost as compared to tablets.
- ❖ Stability concerns with compounds susceptible to hydrolysis.

In a single step, softgels are created, filled, and sealed. The manufacturing process typically continues day and night until the entire lot of a particular product is produced. This leads to a manufacturing environment that is open 24 hours a day, seven days per week.

Oval, oblong, and circular Softgel forms are the most common for oral medicinal preparations. A number that depicts the Softgel's notional capacity in minims (1 cc 14 16.23 minims) is used to indicate its size. For instance, 8.5 to 11.0 minimal fills of fill formulation can be used to fill an 11-oblong Softgel.

With the right die design, softgels can be produced in any shape with a plane of symmetry and any size (to hold up to 25 ml). In each form category, smaller-sized Softgels are preferred, with oval being the most popular shape, according to a recent survey.

DESCRIPTION

The Softgel (Fig. 1) is a one-piece, hermetically sealed capsule with a liquid or semisolid fill instead of an air or gas bubble. Numerous other types of vehicles may be used as fill materials, which may also take the form of a suspension or a solution. Although the Softgels may be clear or opaque, it is customary to employ a clear shell—either naturally amber or one that is dyed clear—only when the fill is also a clear solution. Gelatin, plasticizer, and water historically make up the majority of the shell in the completed product. Recently, non-gelatin materials including starch and carrageenan have been produced into shells for use in Softgel applications. To achieve enteric release of the encapsulated content, softgels may be coated with suitable enteric coating agents, such as cellulose acetate phthalate.

Softgels are widely employed in various medicinal, cosmetic, and dietary products due to their unique qualities and benefits. Oral dose forms, chewable Softgels, suppositories, and topical treatments are the main medicinal applications.

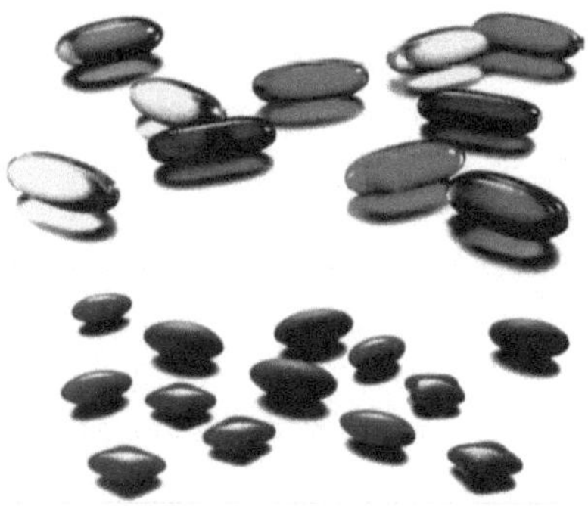

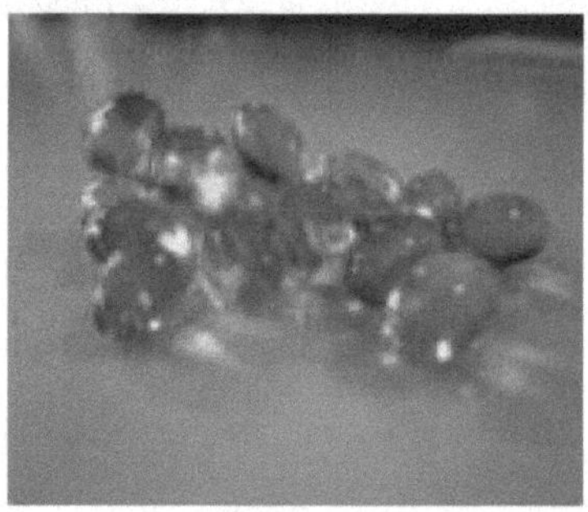

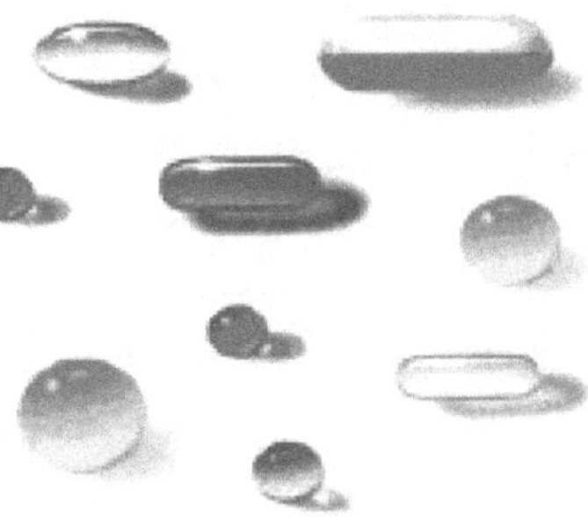

Fig. 1: Examples of Softgels.

FORMULATION DEVELOPMENT

The concepts of softgel formulation will be covered in this part, along with fill and shell formulations made of gelatin.

Shell Formulation

Gelatin has traditionally been used as the polymer base for the shell of softgels. The most popular types of gelatin come from cow sources. In the literature, gelatins made from chicken, fish, or other sources have been mentioned as alternatives to bovine and porcine gelatin. However, due to their limited availability, they have not yet attracted significant economic interest. Plasticizer, water, materials that affect the intended appearance (colorants and/or opacifiers), and, occasionally, flavors and/or preservatives are added in addition to the base polymer. A shell buffer (sodium phosphate dibasic) is also necessary for starch carrageenan. Softgel capsules can also include enteric or delayed release coatings if necessary. The following provides a full explanation of the roles, varieties, and quantities of ingredients used most frequently in creating Softgel shell compositions.

Gelatin

Typically 40–50% of the wet gel formulation for softgels based on gelatin can be either Type A (acid treated) or Type B (alkali processed) gelatin. Based on manufacturing expertise and compatibility with other constituents (both active and inert) in the softgel, the type of gelatin used in a given softgel formulation is chosen. The source of collagen, extraction technique, pH, heat history, and electrolyte content all play a significant role in determining the physicochemical characteristics of gelatin.

This is because gelatin has the following fundamental qualities: It is a good film-forming substance, producing a strong, flexible film; It is readily soluble in biological fluids at body temperature; It is widely used in foodstuffs; It is approved for use internationally.

The strength of the gelatin films comes from their homogenous structural design.

Gelatin Production Process

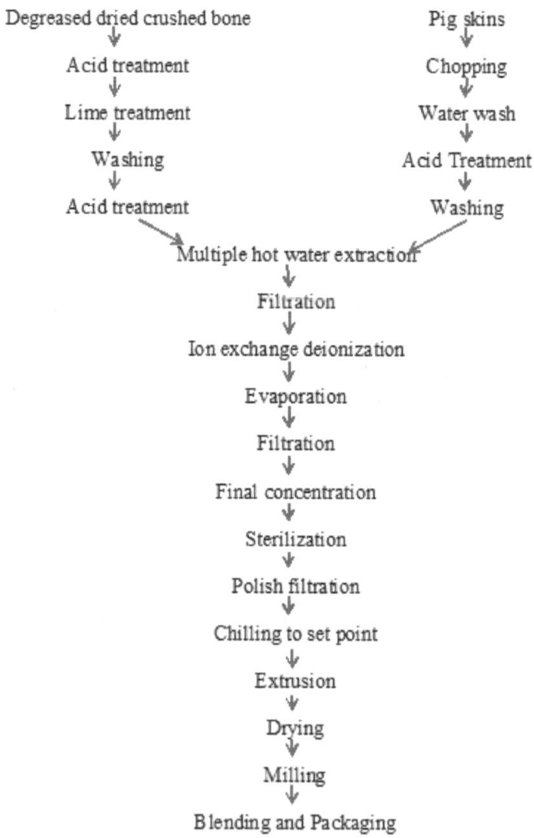

Plasticizers

The Softgel shell is made flexible and elastic using plasticizers. If the fill has no impact, the ratio of plasticizer to shell polymer determines the hardness of the shell. Plasticizers, which can be glycerine, sorbitol, or propylene glycol separately or in combination, typically make about 20–30% of the wet gel composition. It is also possible to utilize a variety of unique sugar combinations containing sorbitol anhydrides, which are offered by excipients vendors. The amount and kind of plasticizer used define the final product's hardness and may have an impact on the Softgel's physical and chemical stability, as well as its capacity to dissolve or disintegrate. The selection of plasticizers takes into account the fill formulation, processing (drying) time, and desired Softgel properties such as hardness, appearance, handling characteristics, stability, and even the target market region.

Water

In order to ensure optimal processing during gel preparation and Softgel encapsulation, water typically makes up 30 to 50 percent of wet gel formulations. After encapsulation, extra water is carefully dried out of the Softgels, bringing the equilibrium water level down to typically less than 10%.

Colorants/opacifiers

In the wet gel formulation, colorants and opacifiers are normally utilized in small amounts. To achieve the appropriate color, tint, or hue for product identification, a broad variety of colorants including FD&C and D&C water-soluble dyes, certified lakes, pigments, and vegetable colors have been included into Softgel shells alone or in combination. To lessen the contrast with the seams, it is generally recommended that the color of the capsule shell be the same as or darker than the fill material.

Sometimes an opacifier is added to the Softgel shell to create an opaque shell for suspension fills or to safeguard chemicals that are light-sensitive. The most popular opacifiers are those using titanium dioxide. It is often necessary to add flavors to the Softgel shell, such as ethyl vanillin and essential oils, in order to mask any potentially offensive substances that may be present inside the Softgel.

Fill Formulation

Active substances that are prepared as a suspension or micro emulsion pre-concentrate can be administered using softgels.

There are two types of large groups of liquids that can be enclosed inside Softgels: water-miscible liquids and water-immiscible liquids.

Water-miscible liquids include non-ionic surfactants like polysorbates and polyethylene glycols (PEG). The most widely utilized PEG grades are those with low molecular weights (like PEG 400), as they are liquid at room temperature. Other water-miscible liquids such propylene glycol, ethanol, and glycerine may also be used in small quantities (up to 5–10%).

Water-immiscible liquids comprise ethers, esters, high molecular weight organic acids, certain alcohols, aliphatic, aromatic, and chlorinated hydrocarbons, as well as vegetable and aromatic oils.

Comprise ethers, esters, high molecular weight organic acids, certain alcohols, aliphatic, aromatic, and chlorinated hydrocarbons, as well as vegetable and aromatic oils.

Low molecular weight water-soluble and volatile organic chemicals, such as certain alcohols, acids, ketones, and esters; water (over 5%); emulsions (whether oil in water or water in oil); extreme pH-valued liquids; and aldehydes are liquids that are likely to cause issues after encapsulation.

It is possible to construct medications into suspensions and encapsulate them if they are not adequately soluble in a solvent or combination of solvents. Different problems need different solutions for suspension formulations. To lessen the possibility of particle size or polymorphism changes during the shelf life, drug solubility in excipients should be kept to a minimal. Additionally, drug particle size needs to be regulated to improve process repeatability and to lessen the detrimental impact on bioavailability for medications that are poorly water-soluble.

For the purposes of equipment requirements for capsulation and suspension homogeneity, insoluble medicines should have particles that are 180 mm in size or smaller. Paraffin wax, beeswax, and hydrogenated vegetable oil are examples of suspending agents for water immiscible vehicles, while solid glycol esters are an example for water miscible vehicles (such as higher molecular weight PEG). To encourage wetting of the components and/or fill dispersion in vivo, surfactants like polysorbates are frequently added to the dispersion.

PRODUCT DEVELOPMENT

This section will outline the normal step-by-step procedure for creating softgels. The steps typically include fill formulation development, shell compatibility, prototype development (lab scale encapsulation), experimental batch manufacture (process development), and clinical supply. The process is then reviewed for performance, along with specialized formulation approaches to improve pharmacokinetic performance, to produce the final product.

Fill Formulation Development

A positive displacement pump is utilized in the Softgel process for fill dosing. These pumps can dose a formulation with a reasonably wide range of viscosities (up to 10,000 cps or more), but there are a number of additional variables that could influence the dosage, most notably the rheological properties. The fill liquid is usually a medication solution or suspension (rather than both in one capsule), and it is usually made to fit inside the smallest Softgel while still maintaining appropriate levels of chemical and physical stability, therapeutic efficacy, and production efficiency. The best option is typically a solution since it may help lessen the detrimental effects of medication particle dispersion on bioavailability.

The problem for solution formulations is often to create a solution that is stable enough to remain in solution during manufacture and shelf life, yet concentrated enough to generate a Softgel size capable of meeting requirements for patient compliance and economics.

Identifying the drug's solubility in a variety of solvents that are acceptable to the pharmaceutical industry is the first step in creating a solution that contains Softgel. The solvents are chosen based on their regulatory acceptability and known compatibility with Softgel dosage forms after the solubility has been established. Typical examples of excipient kinds are as follows:

Co-solvents, Hydrophilic surfactants, Lipophilic surfactants, Hydrophilic solvents, Lipophilic materials

Although it could be essential to combine different solvents to achieve the desired in vitro or in vivo properties and to provide good physical stability, solvents that offer the medicine with a sufficient level of solubility can be chosen. Make sure the fill solution is strong enough to survive the expected dynamic changes that occur within the first 72 hours following encapsulation if the medication solution is poorly water-soluble. This is due to the components' mobility within the Softgel both during and after encapsulation, which does not happen to the same amount in other "dry" dosage forms (water, plasticizers, medicines, etc.). To guarantee that a durable fillformulation is obtained, it is crucial to conduct moisture, plasticizer challenge, and temperature cycling experiments.

The solubility of the medication in a variety of pharmaceutically acceptable solvents is also evaluated for Softgels containing suspension fills, and excipients in which the drug displays little to no solubility are subsequently chosen. For these formulations to adequately suspend the medication during processing, viscosity enhancers are typically needed. This is essential for preserving medication homogeneity while it is being manufactured.

For the optimal manufactureability, the viscosity enhancer's type and concentration are tuned. The fill material should ideally set somewhat after encapsulation to lessen the effects of long-term migration brought on by gravity. To support proper process development, suspension formulations should be created around medications with controlled particle sizes. Dissolution technique creation is a crucial task for softgel suspension formulations and calls for specialist attention to help ensure accurate interpretation.

Shell Compatibility

Testing the shell formulation's compatibility with the fill formulation is a crucial step in the development process. If the fill is not properly matched to the right shell formulation, a number of issues could arise. These can be seen either right away following encapsulation or after the extended storage period mentioned before. Shell compatibility testing has historically been done with fill material and swatches or samples of gel ribbons. Choosing if it is even possible to evaluate shell compatibility without ever manufacturing Softgels is one of the obstacles for Softgel development. It is advisable to do an encapsulation experiment as soon as possible because of this. This job may be carried out utilizing lab scale equipment to make it simpler and more affordable.

Prototype Development (Lab Scale Encapsulation)

One of the distinguishing characteristics of Softgel manufacturing has always been the fact that all of the manufacturing encapsulating equipment was created with mass production in mind. The minimal batch size for such machines was approximately 2.5–5 L, depending on the anticipated yield and capsule quality, even though this served to lessen the likelihood of scale-up problems.

Cardinal Health just began offering lab scale machinery that can make capsules with as little as 100 cc of fill liquid. Using the same encapsulation technique as large-scale equipment, it is now possible to manufacture first-time Softgels in a laboratory setting and create prototypes to test whether the Softgel dosage form is practical for a given medicine. Due to the fact that the air-filled capsule method is a dry procedure and cannot accurately simulate the wet capsule method, this technology renders the use of air-filled capsules to conduct compatibility studies obsolete.

Process Development

A viable manufacturing procedure that will enable the effective manufacture of the trial batch materials required for regulatory and clinical studies must be created when potential fill and shell formulations have been discovered at the laboratory scale. Such process development entails choosing the right tools and examining crucial processing variables, including the order of addition, temperature, mixing environment, and speed

Later process ranging and validation studies will benefit greatly from the information gathered from these development batch investigations. To improve the drying process and the stability of the final product, for instance, the fill moisture and hardness of the capsules will be evaluated during the drying phases. The drying profile of a Soft gel product is shown in Fig. 2.

Clinical Supply

Clinical batches will be produced in accordance with the requirements for clinical research (whether Phase I, II, or III). To guarantee that the process is reliable when the registration batch is manufactured, process development studies should be properly coordinated.

Product Performance Review/Preparation for Process Validation

A product review should be conducted at the conclusion of the product development phase and before process validation to make sure that the development is complete and that the various manufacturing processes can pass process validation. Prior to undertaking process validation (e.g., logo printing process development), preferably at full scale, any holes in the development process may be further explored and addressed at this time. To demonstrate that the product is acceptable at both the upper and lower process ranges, it is desirable to create two or more process challenge batches. This makes it more likely that validation will be effective.

METHOD OF MANUFACTURE

Softgels have been utilized as a medicine delivery technique since the 1830s. Both the hand-dipping method and the plate-press method were used in early manufacturing.

Individual empty Softgel shells were made using the hand-dipping technique, and they were then filled using a syringe or a dropper. The plate-press method required pressing two sheets of wet gelatin together between two molds as a batch procedure. Gelatin sheet depressions were created by the molds, which were afterwards filled with active fill. Gelatin sheets were pressed together with fill material sandwiched between them after a second gelatin sheet was placed on top of the first. The top and bottom sheets of gelatin were cemented together by the pressure of the plate dies, which also cut out the individual Softgels for later drying. Almost all Softgels sold today are produced utilizing the rotary die method. The production method and equipment have advanced significantly over time, yet the fundamental manufacturing principle has mostly remained constant. The gel mass and the fill material are produced by two separate processes that frequently happen simultaneously. The encapsulation procedure that creates wet Softgels brings both together.

The components for the gelatin shell are combined and then heated under vacuum to create the wet gel mass (gelatin, plasticizer, water, colorants and sometimes opacifiers, flavours, and preservatives). The encapsulation machine produces two distinct ribbons, each about 6 inches wide, by casting molten gel mass onto chilled drums after flowing through heated transfer tubes. Throughout the manufacturing process, the ribbons' thickness (typically 0.02-0.04 in.) is meticulously monitored and verified at regular intervals. The gel ribbons go via rollers that maintain the ribbons' proper alignment and lubricate both of their surfaces. Each gel ribbon makes up one of the Softgel's two halves. Two separate color gel ribbons are used to create two-toned Softgels. The production of active fill ingredients happens independently from the mass production of gel. Both the viscosity of all fillers and the suspended material's particle size are crucial variables that are set during development and monitored during manufacturing.

Using the two gel ribbons and the fill material seen in the following fig. 2, softgels are created during the encapsulation phase of the process.

2 Lubricated gel ribbons are fed between two counter-rotating dies that have matching pockets on their surface that are the right size and shape to act as molds for creating the Softgels. Additionally, the die pockets seal the Softgel's two sides and separate the created Softgel from the leftover gel ribbon. Encapsulation is followed by the rapid separation of the softgels from the ribbons. After that, a tumble dryer is used to start the drying process for the Softgels. The wedge is positioned between the ribbons and the revolving dies. The wedge performs three distinct tasks during encapsulation.

To ensure that melting (welding) of the two gel ribbons occurs when the ribbons are forced together between the dies; it warms the gel ribbons initially near to the gel-sol transition temperature.

A positive displacement pump delivers fill material to each of the die pockets, and the wedge is a component of the system that distributes that material.

Finally, the wedge eliminates air from the seal produced between the shells and fill material by acting as a sealing surface against the ribbons in combination with the lubricant. This prevents air from entering the final product. The formulation of the gel mass contains too much water to produce the gel mass and create the gel ribbons effectively. To produce a finished product that will be strong enough to endure additional processing, packaging, and shipping, as well as exhibit good long-term physical stability, Softgels must be dried after encapsulation. Two stages of drying take place. The Softgels are tumbled in air that is controlled for temperature and humidity during their initial drying process in a rotating basket dryer. It is meant to remove enough water so that the capsules are solid enough to endure tray drying without significantly deforming the shape due to gravity. This method removes about half of the surplus water. When the Softgels are spread out in a single layer on shallow trays during the secondary drying step, the remaining surplus water is drained away. Air may circulate around the Softgels and through the rack thanks to the way the trays are made and stacked. The process of secondary drying continues under regulated temperature and humidity settings until the desired degree of capsule hardness and/or fill moisture is reached. Depending on the size of the Softgel and the composition of the shell and fill, complete drying can take anywhere between three days and three weeks. The Softgels are put into bulk holding containers to stop further drying once they have reached the specified drying end point. Several further processes, such as cleaning, off-line printing, checking, and packaging, could be carried out at this stage.

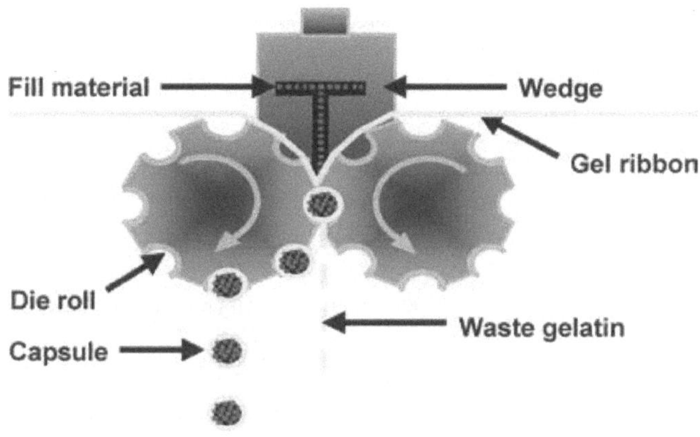

Fig. 2: Softgel encapsulation process

THERAPEUTIC PERFORMANCE

The Softgel dosage form, whose precise formulation relies on the intended pharmacokinetic enhancement, can improve the pharmacokinetic performance of pharmaceuticals. Faster and more thorough absorption are the two most frequent requests. The medicine should be dosed in solution in both situations and should be designed to stay in solution after being dispersed in gastrointestinal media, maybe as a nano-emulsion. It is necessary for the drug to be in solution in a mixture of oils, surfactants, co-surfactants, and perhaps co-solvents when creating nano-emulsion pre-concentrates for Softgel encapsulation.

PRODUCT QUALITY CONSIDERATIONS

Ingredient Specifications

The first specification and control measure used to assess the quality of the final product is assuring acceptable excipients and active ingredient quality. Excipient testing assures compliance with regulatory requirements as well as those established during the formulation of the fill material and/or shell. Limiting values for trace contaminants particularly peroxides, aldehydes, certain metals, and ionic salts, are included in this list. These contaminants can cause cross-linking of gelatin, potential dissolution issues, or unwanted changes in the product's appearance over time. In order to ensure that the gelatin meets current United States Pharmacopeia (USP) specifications as well as additional controls for particle size, viscosity, and bloom strength—all of which are crucial for both the manufacturing process and the stability of the finished product—it is important to note that gelatin is the main ingredient for the shell and is present in higher quantities than other excipients. To guarantee stable product appearance during storage, further criteria are required, such as the proportion of particular ionic components. Additionally, depending on the formulation and target market for the finished product, it is crucial to specify or limit additional gelatin features, such as color or even the source of the gelatin (bovine, porcine, bone, or hide).

In-Process Testing

While the Softgel production process is in the encapsulation stage, a number of tests are regularly carried out. These involve calculating the weight of the fill and shell, as well as measuring the thickness of the seals on the Softgels themselves. During the drying process, measurements of fill moisture and/or hardness are made, and the results are utilized to establish the drying end point for each batch. The dimensions of the Softgel, the quantity and type of fill, as well as the outcomes of earlier process development studies, serve as the basis for the specifications for fill weight, shell weight, seam thickness, and drying end points.

Final Product Testing

The batch is examined and a sample taken for the last product-release test after the Softgels has finished all necessary processing stages. Regulatory requirements for the product determine the tests needed for its final release, which often include microbiological testing, active ingredient identification and assay, physical evaluation, fill weight, dissolution or disintegration testing, and dosage consistency.

CAPSULES, HARD

Since its industrial introduction in the United States in the 19th century, hard or two-piece capsules have been manufactured all over the world. Customers choose hard capsules due of their exquisite design and form, which makes them simple to take. Most capsule fills consist of dry powder blends, which are frequently straightforward formulations. Products are given in this shape for a number of reasons, one of which is the minimal tension required during the processing and filling of the components. Due to the small number of variables involved, the formulator is possible to create goods that have the appropriate release characteristics, such as quick, controlled, or customized release. Hard capsules can be filled with a variety of formulations, ranging from dry solids to non-aqueous liquids, giving the formulator the flexibility to use a variety of excipients to accomplish their intended effects. It is possible to construct capsule products so that they transport their active ingredients to the lungs and release them at various locations along the gastrointestinal track.

RAW MATERIALS

Gelatin and Alternative Materials

Collagen is a naturally occurring protein that is found in the skin, bones, and connective tissues of animals. Collagen is used to make gelatin. It is hydrolyzed to become soluble because it is insoluble in water. Its production requires primarily bovine or porcine bones or skins as raw materials. Type A gelatin, which is predominantly made from skins, can be formed by the reaction when the pH is acidic, and type B gelatin, which is produced when the pH is basic (primarily produced from bovine bones). Because it is palatable, soluble at body temperature, forms sturdy thin films, and goes through a gelation process at temperatures just above ambient, gelatin is an excellent material.

Gelatin capsule walls are uniform and extremely strong, and they can easily bear the mechanical strains of the filling and packaging processes. The biggest disadvantage of using gelatin is that it contains water, which gives the film a plasticizer. When water is lost, their characteristics change, making them brittle and unsuitable for hygroscopic compositions. If they are not stored properly, they will undergo these changes. They cannot be filled with compounds that are moisture-sensitive. There are consumer criteria for a capsule of vegetable origin in some markets. The main challenge in developing a gelatin alternative is to identify a substance that gels similarly to gelatin so that the same manufacturing equipment and procedures can be applied.

Since 1990, a number of polymers—including hypromellose, pullulan, chitosan, and pondac—have been suggested for use in the production of capsules. The reason hypromellose has been the most successful is that it solves the issue of capsule brittleness when exposed to dry conditions. This flaw affects all alternative polymers that have been suggested to some degree. Hard hypromellose capsules are similar to gelatin capsules in appearance but differ in other ways. Their key benefit is that they have far lower moisture contents, and even if this is taken away, they still keep their mechanical strength.

Gelatin capsules with 5% Polyethylene glycol (PEG) 4000 added as an extra plasticizer are also made. Compared to regular gelatin capsules, they have better physical qualities and can lose more moisture before they start to crumble.

CAPSULE MANUFACTURE

A dipping procedure is used to make gelatin capsules. A concentrated solution of gelatin or another suitable polymer is prepared first in hot demineralized water to begin the procedure. To release air bubbles that have become trapped, this solution is put under low pressure. 20–30 L of this solution are taken in small aliquots. Preservatives, process aids such disodium lauryl sulfate solution, colorants, either soluble dye solutions or suspensions of pigments, and water to control the viscosity are all added to this. The finished solution contains 25–30 weight percent gelatin. The capsule manufacturing device is then given this solution.

The rooms housing the manufacturing equipment are ventilated with filtered air, kept at a temperature of 22–25°C and relative humidity of 40–45%. The most often utilized machines are separated into two mirror images of one another along their midline and are roughly 12m long and 3m high. The machines are split into a top level and a lower level along their length. On the left side of the machine, the caps are manufactured, and on the right, the bodies. The gelatin solutions are kept in jacketed hoppers that regulate temperature. They are then fed into the capsule-forming apparatus, also referred to as a dip pan or dip pot. This is an oblong, stainless steel-jacketed vessel with a box in the middle. Pumping the gelatin solution into the box causes it to overflow the edge, keeping the height constant. A row of 30 stainless steel mold pins is set on steel bars. Bar sets are held in a mechanism that a cam controls and can rise and lower. The gelatin solution, which is at 50–55°C, is lowered into the mold pins, which are at 22–22°C. On the mold, the gelatin forms a gel right away. The excess gelatin drips off as the molds are gradually elevated. The amount the mold collects is inversely proportional to the viscosity. The amount of gelatin that is picked up increases with the viscosity of the gelatin solution, As a result, the viscosity of the solution is employed to regulate the gelatin film's thickness. A blob of gelatin forms on the end of the mold as it breaks the surface. The sets of bars are moved from the machine's bottom to its top level while being rotated to uniformly distribute the film over the end of the mold pin.

By the time the molds are transferred to the machine's upper level, the gelatin film has fully dried. Bars are mechanically transported through a number of drying kilns in groups. These are exposed to air that has been carefully managed for temperature and humidity. The bars are moved to the lower level and pushed back toward the machine's front as they approach the machine's conclusion. The moisture content of the gelatin films has been lowered from 70% at dipping to roughly 16 wt% when the bars come out of the drying kilns. Prior to being dipped once more, the molds, which had been warmed at the beginning of the drying process, had returned to machine room temperature.

The cap and body parts are attached once the dry gelatin films have been taken from the mold pins and cut to the appropriate lengths. Pairs of bars, one with bodies and one with caps, are transferred into the middle area of the machine, where this is done automatically. The films are removed from the mold pins and placed into collets by metal jaws that clamp them. The gelatin film is cut as the collets revolve against a knife. The surplus is recycled and sucked away. Transferred to a central connecting block, the two sections are closed to a predetermined length known as the unclosed joined length. Because it would be difficult for the filling machines to separate them, the capsules are not completely closed. When they are closed, the body engages the "prelock" indentations on the cap, creating a strong enough bond to prevent separation during handling.

Hypromellose capsules are made under the same circumstances and to the same standards. The fundamental difference between the two processes is that gelatin solutions quickly transition from the sol to the gel state, whereas their gelling system takes longer to set.

PROCESS OF CAPSULE MANUFACTURING

1. The heated holding hopper on the manufacturing machine receives the prepared gelatin solution.
2. A feed from the holding hopper automatically maintains the solution level.
3. Capsules are created by dipping sets of molds, which are 22°C room temperature, into this solution.
4. By gelling, a film is created on the exterior of each mold.
5. To create a uniformly thick coating, the moulds are gently removed from the solution and rotated as they are moved to the upper level of the machine.
6. After that, groups of "pin bars" are blown over with a sizable volume of regulated humidity air in a series of drying kilns (ovens).
7. The dry films are taken out of the molds, precisely cut to the right length, put together, and the finished capsule is discharged from the machine.

For the beginning of the following cycle, the mould pins are then cleaned and lubricated.

STANDARD FOR EMPTY CAPSULES

Empty capsules are required to meet both analytical and functional criteria. Like all other pharmaceutical preparations, capsules must adhere to cGMP requirements and be constructed from components that meet pharmacopoeial chemical and microbiological criteria. These tests do not, however, reveal whether a capsule would function well on a filling machine. The manufacturers apply a number of functional tests. The lengths and diameters of the caps' and bodies' key dimensions are verified. There will be a very small percentage of cosmetically flawed capsules because production is constant. To evaluate quality from samples, conventional statistical sampling techniques are applied. Users and manufacturers concur on acceptable quality standards (AQL). Depending on how they might affect the filling process or the performance of the capsule, the flaws are grouped into three groups. Each type of fault is given a different AQL.

STORAGE OF EMPTY CAPSULES

To preserve their qualities, capsules should be kept in sealed containers at constant temperatures. The moisture content of empty gelatin capsules ranges from 13% to 16%. In order to preserve the capsule's elasticity and strength, water serves as a plasticizer. If the moisture content exceeds the limitations, they will soften, and if it stays below the limits, they will become brittle. The moisture content of empty hypromellose capsules ranges from 3% to 6%. These capsules can be dried to a moisture content of less than 1% without deteriorating mechanically or becoming brittle. Hard gelatin capsules contain water, but it is insufficient for active bacterial growth since it is tightly bound into the polymer structure.

CAPSULE FILLING

Materials with a wide range of physical qualities can be put inside the two-piece hard capsule. Table 1 displays the many formulations that have been put into capsules. Because of how filling machines handle empty capsules, this is possible.

First, the capsules are positioned so that their bodies are facing downward and that they are all looking in the same direction. The capsules are placed into pairs of bushes; the top bush's aperture at the base only enables the body to pass through, keeping the cap in place. Suction is used to separate the body from the cap. Then, a dosing mechanism is used to deliver material into the open end of the body. To make sure that the self-locking mechanism, which consists of a series of indentations on the cap and body, is correctly engaged, the cap is replaced on the body and the capsule is closed to the correct closed joined length. As a result, filled capsules can be moved and wrapped automatically without splitting. The method by which filling machines measure the dose of material distinguishes them from one another. From bench-scale to high-output industrial scale, and from manual to fully automation, they are offered with a variety of outputs.

Table 1: Formulation types for filling into hard capsules

Dry solids	**Semisolids**	**Liquids**
Powders	Thixotropic mixtures	Oily liquids
Granules	Thermo-softening Mixtures	Non-aqueous solutions and suspensions
Pellets	Pastes	
Tablets		
Capsules		

Types of excipients used in powder filled capsules

Diluents are excipients that are typically concentrated the most in a formulation and provide the necessary bulk when the amount of active substances does not. Examples of diluents include lactose, maize starch, calcium sulfate, etc.

Lubricants and glidants, such as talc and magnesium stearate, that lessen the adherence of powder to metal and enhance flow properties

Wetting agents help poorly soluble medications, like sodium lauryl sulphate, penetrate the water more effectively.

Disintegrants, such as crospovidone and sodium starch glycolate, promote the disruption of the powder mass.

Powder Filling

Dry powder combinations make up the majority of formulations that are put into capsules. Dependent and independent techniques of assessing the dose can be separated into two categories. The independent machines employ a separate instrument, whereas the dependent machines use the capsule body directly to measure the dose of powder. Compared to the literature on tableting, there is less information available on the mechanics of capsule filling. Tablets, as opposed to capsules, are employed in a variety of businesses outside the healthcare industry; hence there have been significantly more workers in the field.

a. **Dependent type** - The first filling devices used in industry were dependent ones. The body of the capsule receives the powder straight from a hopper. Either a vibrating plate or a rotating auger helps the powder to flow. These capsules have a loose fill of powder bulk. The body is overfilled on auger machines; therefore more of the capsule shell's internal capacity is utilized than is the case with automatic independent type machines, leading to larger fill weights. Suction is used to help feed the empty capsules into a pair of doughnut-shaped plates, separating them. Removed and set aside is the upper plate that held the caps. The powder hopper is pushed over the bottom plate holding the bodies after it has been manually moved to a turntable. The bodies' plate rotates beneath the hopper as the auger forces powder into them. The turntable and auger's rotational speeds determine the fill weight. Complete filling of the bodies is the only method to have acceptable fill weight uniformity on these machines. Filling only partially is not an option. A three-roller system for capsule orientation and continuous feeding to a rotating disk assembly, where the capsules are separated, filled, and re-joined, are features of a fully automatic rotary auger-filling machine. Other automatic dependent filling uses vibration instead of augers to liquefy the powder for filling into the bodies as they pass beneath the hopper. Only dense, freely flowing material can be used in this technique.

I. **Independent type** - The majority of industrial automatic machines are of the independent kind, which compresses the measured quantity of powder to create a plug. The dosing tube (or dosator) and the dosing disc and tamping finger are two different sorts of mechanisms.

II. **Dosing tube** - The most popular kind is the dosage tube. A moving piston that controls the dosing volume and provides force to form the plug inside a tube is used to form the plug. While the higher output machines rotate, the lower output machines move intermittently. Because a large portion of the machine cycle is spent indexing the components, intermittent machines tend to put more strain on the powder than rotary machines because there is less time to create the plug. As a result, formulations for these machines frequently call for more lubricant. Because the fill weight may be changed across a wide range by making a simple adjustment to the piston position, these machines are incredibly adaptable. The rotary machines can be connected to check weighing equipment that can automatically adjust the fill weight and enable them to run unattended.

III. **Dosing disc and tamping finger machines** - The plug-forming processes used by the tamping finger and dosing disc devices are similar but distinct. This includes up to six sets of machined holes and serves as the powder hopper's foundation. Above the powder hopper, there is a holder with sets of stainless steel tamping fingers that match the disc's holes. The motion of these devices is irregular. The tamping fingers are dropped into the powder bed once the machine has indexed and the turret is still. The fingers are positioned at various levels, and as they enter the plate, they cause the powder in the cavities to solidify into plugs. As a result, rather than in a single movement as it is on dosator machines, the plug is formed by a series of tamps. For each size of capsule, a variety of thicknesses of the dosage discs are created. Therefore, choosing the right disc thickness is crucial because if the fill weight cannot be reached, the machine must be disassembled in order to replace it. With the aid of a straightforward test rig or methodically, by measuring the plug density and strength of a formulation under known compression forces, an Instron tester can be used to choose the ideal disc thickness for a formulation.

Bench-Scale Filling Machines

There are numerous tools available for manually filling small batches of capsules. These normally consist of sets of plastic plates with sets of holes drilled into them that are sized to fit the various sizes of capsules. Torpac Inc. sells a product constructed of stainless steel and other metal alloys that may be autoclaved to assure cleanliness without the risk of distortion. The capsules are manually placed one at a time into the plates or are fed into the plates in groups using a feeding apparatus. The top plate is removed while the bodies are clamped in the lower plate, separating the body from the caps. When the bodies are freed, they rest below the bottom plate's top. The capsules are filled by spreading material over the body plate using a spatula to create powder or pellets.

Instrumented Filling Machines

Contrary to tableting machines, instrumented capsule filling equipment is not commonly used. This is partially due to the fact that less fundamental research has been done; quantifying the modest forces (1-100 N) used to produce and eject plugs presents an inherent challenge, and the powder bed is less regulated than in a tablet die. The majority of research that have been published have been done using intermittent motion dosing tube devices. To gauge the effort required for plug generation, strain gauges have been attached to the piston and linear variable displacement transducers (LVDTs) to the system's moving components. On an instrumented dosing disc and tamping finger machine, just two groups have used it. The issue with these machines is that thorough instrumentation would be challenging because the plug is created at up to five separate positions. To get around some of the issues that arise with mounting instrumentation on real machines, capsule filling machine stimulators have been developed. The movement of the dosing elements on rotary operating machines is the main issue. One option was to build a rig that rotated the powder hopper around the dosator to simulate a machine running and utilize a machine turret with a single dosator that was held stationary. A standard stimulator for an intermittent motion dosator machine has been created that can monitor the radial compression force in addition to the axial compression and ejection forces. This has been utilized to research the elastic and consolidation characteristics of excipients. The investigation of plug production at low stresses was conducted using a tablet compaction simulator, and the findings were examined using conventional tableting physics.

Dry Solid Filling

Automatic filling devices can automatically fill capsules with granules, pellets, and tablets. These techniques of product preparation can be used to alter the rate at which active substances release, to separate incompatible elements, or to densify a product to reach the fill weight required for a certain size of capsule. There are direct and indirect types of filling equipment that can be utilized for pellets and granules. In the former, the body is given pellets and granules until it is entirely satisfied. Indirect machines have modified dosators that are either filled as they are pushed up through the material bed or employ suction to hold the material in the tube during transfer. Various chambers with movable plates are used by other indirect machines to provide a variable volume in which to measure the material. Following measurement, pellets and grains are transported to the capsule bodies either by gravity or with the use of air pressure. Systems that can handle both single and multiple additions fill tablets into capsules. To ensure that the right quantities of tablets have been dosed, they feature mechanical or electrical sensing devices. These formulations' physical characteristics are comparable. Each type should ideally not be friable; film coating is typically present on tablets. Capsules are loaded with a variety of pills. The tablets are typically convex in shape and have diameters that make it easy to insert them into the body and provide enough room for them to stay upright.

Liquid Filling

Machines that can fill capsules with liquid have been produced by all the main machine makers. Liquid fills can be divided into two categories: formulations that are liquefied solely for the filling process using heat or shear stress, and formulations that are non-aqueous solutions and suspensions. The capsules must be sealed after filling if the mixture is mobile at room temperature. Volumetric pumps are used to measure the dosage of the substance; hence the fill uniformity is typically better than what can be obtained with a typical powder filling machine. Coefficients of variation in fill weight that are less than 1.0% are frequently possible. This figure will be influenced by the liquid's physical characteristics, particularly its viscosity. There are filling devices available that can work with materials with viscosities ranging from 0.1 to 20 Pa. Comparable powder filling devices run primarily at faster speeds than liquid filling machines. This occurs because it takes longer for the liquid to move through a smaller opening than it does for a powder. The rates are normally between 50 and 66% of the rated output of a machine that fills powder in the same size.

Capsule Fill Capacity

The physical dimensions of a hard capsule, the kind of formulation, and the dosing mechanism on the filling equipment all affect the fill capacity. Historically, the fill weight of powders has been determined by multiplying a powder density number by the capacity of the capsule as supplied by the capsule manufacturers. This measurement of the capsule body capacity was made using actual data from the time when pills were manually filled in pharmacies. The connection, when the volume number is multiplied by the tapped bulk density (TBD) of the powder mixture, provides a fairly accurate forecast for machine filling. The machine-dosing methods maintain the link. Dependent machines are only able to pack the powder into the bodies of the capsules at densities lower than the TBD of the fill, even if they can fill the entire interior volume of the capsule. The interior diameter and length of the capsule must be less than the dimensions of the plugs for them to fit inside of a closed capsule, which are created by independent machines capable of applying a larger compressive force to the powder. As a result, even if the plug's density will be higher than the fill's TBD, the machines cannot fill the entire interior capsule volume.

Pellet and granular filling follow the same packing regulations. The increase in voidage brought on by large particles in a small diameter tube makes the particle size crucial. To obtain equal fill weights, the particles' equivalent size should be smaller the smaller the capsule size. To avoid product leakage, the liquid fill volume of capsules is limited; it should not be greater than 90% of the body volume.

Capsule Sealing

For the purpose of stopping liquid leakage from capsules, many techniques have been suggested. Gelatin banding has been found to be the most effective technique. Around the center of the filled capsule, two bands of gelatin solution are placed. To avoid the gelatin shells losing moisture and becoming brittle, this band is dried using air at ambient temperatures. The band's color-changing capability enables a more complex visual for product branding. The Food and Drug Administration's (FDA) "Tamper-Evident Packaging Requirements for Over-the-Counter Human Drug Products" are met by this band when it comes to tamper-evident sealed capsules.

Multiple Contents

There are automatic filling machines that can have multiple product-dosing mechanisms. As a result, mixtures of materials, such as a powder and a semisolid formulation or a powder and a tablet, can be put into the same capsule. For many forms, the same formulation guidelines apply. The formulator can accomplish particular objectives in terms of product stability and release types by the combination of components.

Difficulties in filling capsules

1. **Deliquescent or filling capsules** -A gelation capsule contains water that is removed from or absorbed by a hygroscopic medication, making the capsule extremely brittle and causing it to break. Adsorbents like magnesium carbonate are added. If the capsules are contained in firmly sealed glass capsule vials, either heavy magnesium oxide or light magnesium oxide can be used to solve this challenge.
2. **Eutectic mixtures** – Due to the creation of a mixture with a lower melting point than room temperature, certain substances have a tendency to liquefy and produce a pasty mass when combined. Each problematic ingredient is blended with an absorbent separately before being combined and put into capsules for these kinds of chemicals. Kaolin and magnesium oxide are the absorbents employed. Another approach to solving this problem is to combine the ingredients to create a eutectic mixture, which is then added an absorbent such as magnesium carbonate or kaolin.
3. **Addition of inert powders** – When a very little amount of the drug needs to be placed within capsules and it is not feasible to do so, an inert substance or diluent is added to the powder to increase its volume. This is simple to load into capsules.
4. **Use of two capsules** – Some manufacturers split the formulation's incompatible elements by packing one of the ingredients into a smaller capsule. After which

inserting this tiny capsule into the larger capsule holding the remaining formulation components.

5. **Filling of granular powder** - Because they are not compressible and flow out of the capsules as soon as they are lifted from the pile of powder into which they were punched, some powders that lack adhesiveness and the majority of granular powders are difficult to fill in the capsule by punch method. In order to get over this problem, the non-adhesive powder needs to be moistened with alcohol and the granular powder needs to be ground into powder before being put into capsules.

FORMULATION

Powder Properties

In order to create plugs at low compression forces, powder formulations for capsule filling must have appropriate flow characteristics, be non-adhesive, and be sufficiently cohesive. They also need to release the active ingredient in the desired way and be stable. In order to create formulations logically, it is necessary to comprehend how the formulation, the filling machine, and the empty capsules interact. A range of tests, from the most basic to the most complicated, can be used to evaluate the powder-filling characteristics on a bench scale. Several articles have successfully correlated powder properties with filling performance by calculating several powder property constants from TBD volumetry. Lu dde-constant Kawakita's and Hausner's ratio was found to be reliable predictors of machine filling performance for various microcrystalline celluloses. Studies on the packing characteristics of binary mixes of variously shaped particles have demonstrated that the Lu dde- Kawakita constant can be used as a gauge for the greatest volume loss. Spherical or needle-shaped particles have a tendency to worsen packing qualities, but lactose monohydrate, an angular particle, and microcrystalline cellulose all increase packing. Following granulation or low compression, the bulk volume variations of powders were investigated using the same methods. This demonstrated that high-shear granulation or machine compression might improve capsule fill weights and that the result was closely proportional to the initial powder qualities. The variety of tissue materials utilized makes it more difficult to fill capsules with powdered herbs. These materials have poor flow characteristics, so it was decided to determine a range of powder property constants in an effort to identify a variable that was connected with filling machine performance. It was discovered that tamp-filling devices could handle a wider range of herbs than dosator devices. Using specially designed rheometers, the flow of powders under active conditions may be measured, and the results can be connected to other powder characteristics. The design of the machine helps the powders flow on the filling machine. The majority of machines feature components that move mechanically, vibrate, or have suction pads to help with flow. Obtaining adequate fill-weight homogeneity is hampered by the material's adhesion to moving elements, especially the dose-measuring apparatuses. It has been demonstrated that a significant consideration is the dosator's surface texture. The surface of the dosing components can be coated with various metal finishes, similar to those used for tablet punches and dies, to lessen adherence.

CAPSULE COATING

Extemporaneous coatings have been applied to improve appearance, mask taste, and stop the drug from dissolving in the stomach (enteric coated products). The majority of capsule coatings require sophisticated formulation expertise and quality control tools often found in production facilities. To prevent the active medication from dissolving before it reaches a specific area of the digestive tract, capsules might be coated. Stearic acid, shellac, casein, cellulose acetate phthalate, and natural and manufactured waxes are examples of materials that are acceptable. The reason for their use is their acid insolubility but alkaline solubility.

a. **Enteric coated capsules** – The enteric coated capsules resist stomach breakdown but crumble in the intestine. Enteric coated pills have essentially replaced them. The following types of medications are eligible for enteric coating:

- ❖ For medications such as amoebicides and anthelmintics that arc designed to work in the intestine, as well as for drugs that irritate the gastric mucosa or are degraded by the gastric juice.
- ❖ Which hinder digestion, such as tannins, silver nitrate, and other heavy metal salts.
- ❖ Which are required to produce delayed action of the drug

Several coating methods may be used and are described below

1. **Beaker flask coating** – Put a tiny bit of the coating substance in the flask and warms it up gradually until it melts. Add a few capsules, turn off the heat, and then twist the flask to begin coating. Continue rotating while adding a few more drops of melted coating material every so often. All that is necessary to prevent the capsules from clumping and adhering together are extremely modest additions.
2. **Dipping** - in a beaker, heat the coating material to the lowest temperature practical. Tweezers can be used to dip individual capsules, let the coating cool, and then repeat the procedure until thick enough layers has formed.

2.9 Spraying - The coating material is prepared and put in a little sprayer along with an alcoholic or ethereal solution. The capsules are arranged on a screen in an area with good ventilation. Very thin coatings of the coating solution are applied, with enough time between coats for drying. Up until a suitable layer is formed, the operation is repeated.

EVALUATION OF CAPSULES

Evaluation of commercial capsules:

1- Content uniformity:

- ✓ 30 capsules are selected and 10 of these are assayed individually.
- ✓ At least 9 of these contain 85 – 115 % of drug and none contain below 75 – 125% of drug.
- ✓ If 1 to 3 of them fall outside of 85 – 115% limits, the remaining 20 capsules
- ✓ are individually assayed and the requirements are met if no few than 27 contain 85 – 115 % of drug and none contain less than 75 – 125 % of drug.

2- Weight Uniformity: This test applies to all types of capsules and it is to be done on 20 capsules.

Method:

1- Weigh an intact capsule.

2- Open the capsule without losing any part of the shell and remove the contents as completely as possible.

3- Weigh the shell.

4- The weight of the contents is the difference between the weighing.

5- Repeat the procedure with a further 19 capsules selected at random.

6- Determine the average weight.

3- Disintegration:

The disintegration test determines whether tablets or capsules disintegrate within a prescribed time when placed in a liquid medium under the prescribed experimental conditions.

Method:

According to the B.P. and applies to hard and soft capsules.

1- Introduce one capsule into each tube and suspend the apparatus in a beaker containing 600 ml water at 37 °C. If hard capsules float on the surface of the water, the discs may be added.

2- Operate the apparatus for 30 minutes; remove the assembly from the liquid.

3-The capsules pass the test if

– No residue remains on the screen of the apparatus or,

– If a residue remains, it consists of fragments of shell or,

– Is a soft mass with no palpable core

– If the disc is used, any residue remaining on its lower surface should only consist of fragments of shell.

4- Dissolution:

- The dissolution test is carried out using the dissolution apparatus official in both the U.S.P. and N.F.

- The capsule is placed in a basket formed from 40-mesh stainless steel fabric.

- A stirrer shaft is attached to the basket, and the basket is immersed in the dissolution medium and caused to rotate at a specified speed.

- The dissolution medium is held in a covered 1000 ml glass vessel and maintained at 37°C ± 0.5°C by means of a suitable constant temperature water bath.

- The stirrer speed and type of dissolution medium are specified in the individual monograph.

MICROENCAPSULATION

The microencapsulation techniques result in tiny particles with sizes ranging from 1 to 1000 m. The terms "microparticle," "microsphere," "microcapsule," and "micromatrix" are all used to describe tiny particles. Although the terms are frequently used synonymously, they can be distinguished in that micromatrices are polymeric matrices in which the encapsulated substances are uniformly distributed while microcapsules are made of one or more core substances (solid or liquid) that are surrounded by a distinct capsule wall.

4.1.1 Representative applications ofmicroencapsulation in the pharmaceutical and biomedical industries include:

1. Taste and odor masking

2. Protection of drugs from the environment
3. Particle size reduction for enhancing solubility of the poorly soluble drugs
4. Sustained or controlled drug delivery
5. Cell encapsulation
6. Separation of incompatible components
7. Conversion of liquids to free flowing solids
8. Targeted release of encapsulated materials

Since it is easily adaptable to many administration strategies, the microparticle system has emerged over the past few decades as an essential component of the controlled drug delivery sectors. In comparison to traditional parenteral formulations, biodegradable polymeric microparticles can offer a variety of benefits, including:

Sustained delivery: Microparticles keep the blood level of a medicine within a therapeutic window for an extended period of time by encapsulating it in a polymer matrix that prevents biological fluid from accessing it until the drug is degraded. By lowering the frequency of administration, toxic side effects can be reduced and patient adherence can be increased.

Local delivery: Microparticles can keep a therapeutically effective concentration at the site of action for a desired amount of time when injected subcutaneously or intramuscularly. The local delivery method eliminates the need to administer drugs systemically in order to achieve local therapeutic effects and potentially lessen associated systemic negative effects. The distribution of local anesthetics has shown to be advantageous using this technique.

Pulsatile delivery: Although burst and pulsatile release isn't thought to be ideal for continuous delivery applications, it works well for the delivery of vaccinations and medicines. Antibiotics that are released in pulses can slow the emergence of bacterial resistance. Initial bursts followed by delayed release pulses can simulate the initial and boost injections in vaccine delivery, respectively.

Classification:

Microcapsules can be classified on three basic categories according to their morphology as follows,

1. Mononuclear
2. Polynuclear and
3. Matrix types

While polynuclear capsules have many cores encased within the shell, mononuclear (core-shell) microcapsules only have the shell around the core. The core material is evenly distributed throughout the shell material in matrix encapsulation.

Microcapsules can have several shells, be mononuclear, or form clusters in addition to these three fundamental geometries.

MATERIALS AND METHODS FOR MICROENCAPSULATION

A basic understanding of the general characteristics of microcapsules, such as the nature of the core and coating materials, the stability and release characteristics of the coated materials, and the microencapsulating processes, are necessary for the preparation of microspheres.

Core Material:

The core material in table 2, which is the particular material that will be coated, might be either liquid or solid in composition. Since the liquid core can contain material that is disseminated and/or dissolved, the composition of the core material can vary. A combination of active ingredients, stabilizers, diluents, receivers, release-rate retardants, or accelerators, can make up the solid core. The capacity to change the composition of the core material offers clear flexibility, and making use of this quality frequently enables successful design and development of the necessary microcapsule features.

Table 2: Core material and its purpose

Core Material	Characteristic Property	Purpose of Encapsulation	Final Product Form
Acetaminophen	Slightly water soluble solid	Taste-masking	Tablet
Activated Charcoal	Adsorbent	Selective sorption	Dry Powder
Liquid crystals	Liquid	Conversion of liquid to solid; stabilization	Flexible film for thermal mapping of anatomy
Potassium chloride	Highly water-soluble solid	Reduced gastric irritation	Capsule
Isosorbidedinitrate	Water-soluble solid	Sustained release	Capsule

Coating Materials:

The final physical and chemical features of the micro capsules are largely determined by the choice of the correct coating material. The coating material must have the ability to produce a layer that is cohesive with the core material, be chemically inert and nonreactive with the core material, and offer the desired coating attributes, such as strength, flexibility, impermeability, optical properties, and stability. There is some room for in situ modification of the coating materials employed in micro encapsulation techniques.

When choosing the ideal microcapsule coating material, the standard coating features such as cohesiveness, permeability, moisture sorption, solubility, stability, and clarity must be taken into account as listed in table 3.

For examples

Table 3: Coating material and its purpose

Water-soluble resins	**Water-insoluble resins**	**Waxes and lipids**	**Enteric resins**
Gelatin	Ethyl cellulose	Paraffin	Shellac
Gum Arabic	Polyethylene	Carnauba	Cellulose acetate phthalate
Starch	Polymethacrylate	Beeswax	Zein
Polyvinylpyrrolidione	Polyamide (Nylon)	Stearic acid	
Carboxymethylcellulose	Cellulose nitrate	Stearyl alcohol	
Hydroxyethylcellulose	Silicones	Glyceryl stearates	

MICROENCAPSULATION TECHNIQUES

Coacervation

One of the early microencapsulation methods was the coacervation technique, which has been applied to numerous consumer goods. This technique relies on the division of a solution of hydrophilic polymer(s) into two phases, which are composed of tiny droplets of a dense phase that is rich in polymer and a liquid phase that is more diluted. Depending on the amount of polymers involved in the creation of the microparticles, coacervation can be classified as simple or complicated.

Simple coacervation

One polymer (such as gelatin, polyvinyl alcohol, or carboxymethyl cellulose) is used in this procedure, and the phase separation can be brought about by circumstances that cause the polymer phase to become desolventized (or dehydrated). A water-miscible non-solvent such as ethanol, acetone, dioxane, isopropanol, or propanol may be added, as well as inorganic salts such sodium sulfate and a change in temperature.

Complex coacervation

Two hydrophilic polymers with opposing charges are used in this procedure. To separate the polymer-rich phase, the total positive charges on one of the polymers are neutralized by the negative charges on the other (Fig. 4). The gelatin-gum Arabic method is the most well-known example. Due to the involvement of electrostatic interactions, the pH of the medium is crucial. For instance, the pH level in the gelatin-gum Arabic combination needs to be below the gelatin's isoelectric point in order for the gelatin to keep its positive charge. These polymer complexes are stabilized by cross-linking with glutaraldehyde after embryonic coacervates develop around the scattered or solid phases.

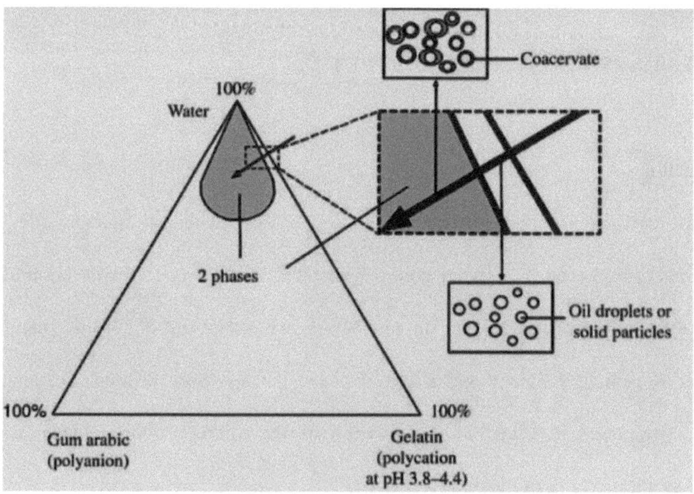

Fig. 4: Phase diagram of complex coacervation.

Emulsion Solidification

From the emulsion of two or more immiscible liquids, microparticles can be created. For instance, to create an oil-in-water (o/w) emulsion, a hydrophobic drug and polymer solution in an organic solvent (oil phase, dispersed phase) is emulsified in an aqueous solution containing an emulsifying agent (water phase, continuous phase). As the solvent is drained away, the drug's polymer-containing particle suspension may solidify. Water-in-oil-in-water (w/o/w for encapsulation of water-soluble drug in water-insoluble polymer), water-in-oil-in-oil (w/o/o for encapsulation of water-soluble drug in water-soluble polymer), or water-in-oil (w/o for encapsulation of water-soluble drug in water-soluble polymer) are the three different types of emulsions. Solid-in-o the emulsion process can be divided into three categories: cross-linking, solvent extraction, and solvent evaporation depending on how the discontinuous droplets are solidified.

Solvent evaporation

Usually, a volatile organic solvent like methylene chloride is used to dissolve the polymer. The polymer solution is combined with drugs or diagnostic agents, either in liquid form or dispersed as tiny solid particles. This mixture is then emulsified in an aqueous solution including an emulsifying agent such poly(vinyl alcohol) (PVA). The resulting emulsion is agitated until the majority of the organic solvent evaporates, leaving solid microparticles that are freeze-dried and can then be washed with water. The emulsion is frequently heated just above the solvent's boiling point to aid in solvent evaporation. For instance, the emulsion is heated to 40°C when methylene chloride (boiling point: 39.8°C) is used as an organic solvent.

Solvent extraction

The solvent evaporation method requires volatile solvents like methylene chloride since it depends on the solvent's high vapour pressure. Otherwise, the solidification process would take too lengthy and produce microspheres with excessive porosity, uneven shape, a loss of payload, or increased polydispersity in the size distribution. In this situation, extraction into the continuous phase can be used to get rid of the comparatively non-volatile solvents. This can be accomplished by using a solvent that is highly soluble in the continuous phase, widening the concentration gap between the continuous and dispersed phases, or mixing in a third solvent to speed up solvent extraction as shown in fig. 5.

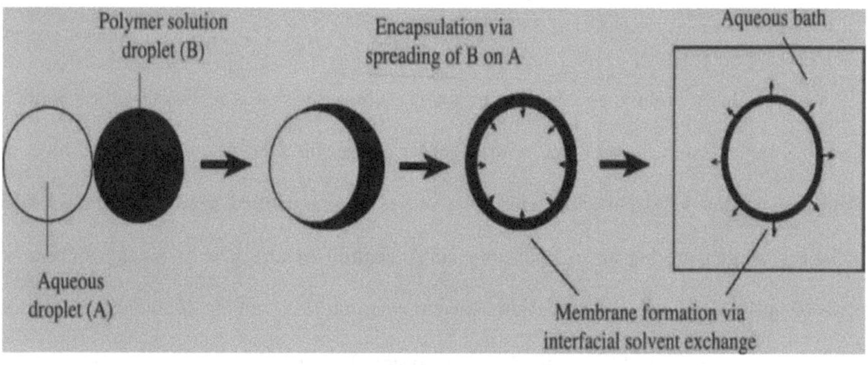

Fig. 5: Microencapsulation based on the solvent exchange method.

Cross-linking method

Many naturally occurring hydrophilic polymers, including gelatin, albumin, starch, dextran, hyaluronic acid, and chitosan, can be solidified through the use of chemical or thermal cross-linking. A w/o emulsion is created by emulsifying the polymer solution in an oil phase that contains an emulsifying agent, such as Span 80. Typically, vegetable oils or oil-organic solvent mixes are used in this process. Although glutaraldehyde is used to cross-link the majority of proteins, its toxicity still poses a challenge in pharmaceutical applications. Alternative cross-linking techniques include heating, introducing counter polyions, or using cross-linking reagents.

Hot-Melt Microencapsulation

After being melted, the polymer is combined with either liquid or solid medicinal components. Under constant stirring, this mixture is heated to 5°C over the polymer's melting point while suspended in an immiscible solvent. The droplets then solidify as the emulsion is cooled below its melting point.

Ionic Gelation/Polyelectrolyte Complexation

Polyelectrolytes are cross-linked during ionic gelation in the presence of multivalent counterions. For instance, stiff gel particles are created when a sodium alginate solution is sprayed into a calcium chloride solution. Polyelectrolyte complexation with polyelectrolytes with opposing charges frequently occurs after ionic gelation. The complexation boosts the mechanical strength of the gel particles by creating a membrane of polyelectrolyte complex on their surface. Polylysine is a common ingredient in calcium alginate gel particles for this function. Chitosan/triphosphate, carboxymethylcellulose/aluminum (or chitosan), k-carrageenan/potassium (or chitosan), pectin/calcium, gelan gum/calcium, and polyphosphazene/calcium are additional polymer systems that can be utilized for ionic gelation (polyelectrolyte complexation) (or polylysine). This technique was created by Lim and Sun to encapsulate cells; in modern times, it is frequently employed to encapsulate both cells and drugs.

Interfacial Polymerization

At the boundary between two immiscible compounds, monomers can polymerize to form a membrane. One illustration is a nylon membrane produced at the interface by the polymerization of two monomers (usually dichloride and diamine). A w/oemulsion is created by combining a non-aqueous phase with surfactant with an aqueous phase with medicines and diamine. The emulsion is then given an extra non-aqueous phase containing acid chloride to enable interfacial polymerization. You can stop polymerization by adding too much non-aqueous phase.

Spray Drying

The closed-system, one-step process of spray drying can be used on a wide range of materials. A suitable (either aqueous or non-aqueous) solvent containing polymer components is used to dissolve or suspend the medication. When a solution or suspension is atomized and placed in a drying chamber, heated carrier gas dries the atomized droplets, resulting in the formation of microparticles. The outcome of the spray drying procedure significantly depends on the characteristics of the material: The product parameters, such as particle size, yield, temperature load, and solvent content, can be affected by the instrument settings, including inlet temperature, feed rate, spray air flow, and aspirator flow. Trial and error is typically used to optimize these settings.

Spray Desolvation

Spray desolvation entails misting a polymer solution onto a liquid that is desolving. For instance, spraying a PVA solution into an acetone bath can produce microparticles. PVA precipitates to create solid microparticles when the polymer solvent (water) is extracted into acetone in this instance. Another instance of this is the encapsulation of bovine serum albumin (BSA) in poly (lactic-co-glycolic acid) (PLGA). The medication was micronized, suspended in a PLGA-acetone solution, then ultrasonically atomized into an ethanol bath.

The cryogenic solvent extraction method is a variation of this technique. Drugs are dissolved or disseminated in the PLGA and methylene chloride-based polymer phase. This drug-polymer solution is atomized on a bed of liquid nitrogen-freezed ethanol. Following their contact with the liquid nitrogen, the microscopic droplets sink into the ice-covered layer of ethanol. The frozen micro-droplets start to dissolve into the ethanol that is thawing as the temperature rises. The methylene chloride in the polymer phase thaws and is then gently drained into ethanol, resulting in the formation of solidified microparticles. A microparticle formulation for human growth hormone was made using this method (hGH). In the formulation stage before encapsulation, hGH is combined with zinc to create an insoluble Zn-hGH complex. This complex's encapsulation helped to stabilize hGH both during the production process and once the microspheres had been hydrated. This formulation's in vivo investigation showed a decreased Cmax and a prolonged serum level for weeks with a biocompatibility similar to the protein solution. The hGH formulation created using this technique (ProLease) was sold as an injectable suspension to be taken once or twice a month.

Spray Coating

In spray coating, solid medication core particles are rotated in a coating chamber while the coating material is sprayed on top of them. Usually, this technique is applied to coating tables or capsules.

Fluid-bed coating (Air-suspension technique)

Fluid-bed procedures include the top, tangential, and bottom spray techniques. The bulk density of the granules generated by the top-spray granulator method is typically lower than that possible by other granulation processes because the coated granules typically have a porous surface and an interstitial void area. A rotating-disk approach, also known as a tangential-spray coating method, produces a product with a higher bulk density but some interstitial void space by combining centrifugal, high-density mixing and the effectiveness of fluid-bed drying. Particles produced with this technique are less friable and have a more spherical form. In the Wurster method (bottom spray), a solution of wall materials is sprayed on to the fluidized solid core particles from the bottom of the fluidization chamber in a direction parallel to the air stream. The coating solution droplets only travel a short distance before coming into contact with the solid particles because the spraying nozzle is immersed in the airflow and simultaneously spray the coating ingredients into the fluidized particles. As a result, the coating is more homogeneous and the film is applied more uniformly. The air stream lifts the coated particles, and as they are moved away from the nozzle, the air stream dries the coating. The airborne particles rise, settle, and then start the process all over again. Till the necessary film thickness is reached, the cycles are repeated. The uniform coating of particles with a polymeric membrane in a single operation is particularly well suited to the Wurster process.

Pan Coating

Pan coating can contain rather big particles. The size of the solid particles must be greater than 600 mm in order to use this technique for successful coating. This is a common technique for coating candy in sugar. This technique involves ladling warm sucrose solution over a revolving drum that contains core materials (like candy). The rotation increases the syrup's surface area, which helps the water vaporize by coating the cores with an even thin layer of syrup. The sugar hardens and coating the cores as the water evaporates. Perforated pans are utilized for medicinal items, and the coating solution—typically an aqueous solution—is sprayed over the rotating cores.

Supercritical Fluid

Utilizing two unique characteristics of supercritical fluids, the relatively new supercritical fluid technology can reduce the need of harsh production environments and organic solvents (i.e., high compressibility and liquid-like density). This process can be roughly divided into two parts: supercritical anti-solvent crystallization (SAS), which uses the fluid as an anti-solvent to cause polymer precipitation, and rapid expansion of supercritical solutions (RESS), which uses the supercritical fluid (such as carbon dioxide) as a solvent for the polymer. The literature includes recent analyses of the supercritical technique for particle generation.

SELECTION OF THE MICROENCAPSULATION METHODS

Different medications cannot all be microencapsulated using the same technique. Understanding the physicochemical characteristics of a medicine is crucial for creating a novel microparticle system for it, as well as selecting an encapsulation technique and polymeric materials that best match those characteristics. The solubility of the medicine in water frequently serves as a useful beginning point for the survey because water is the most commonly employed solvent system. The drug's physical condition may also restrict your options. Table 4 provides a summary of the microencapsulation techniques that have been widely employed for medications with various features.

Table 4: Selection of microencapsulation methods for drugs with different properties

	Water-soluble drugs	**Water-insoluble drugs**
Liquid drugs	w/o/w double emulsion	o/w or o/o emulsion
	w/o/o double emulsion	Coacervation
	w/o emulsion	Spray drying
	Ionic gelation	
	Spray drying	
Solid drugs	Cryogenic solvent extraction method	Coacervation

	s/o/w or s/o/o emulsion	Fluid-bed coating
	Fluid-bed coating	
	Supercritical fluid	

RECENT ADVANCES IN THE MICROENCAPSULATION TECHNOLOGY

A few recent problems with the microencapsulation technique are outlined in this section. Highly interdisciplinary approaches have been used to look for solutions to these problems. This section's final section introduces some recent developments in the field of microencapsulation technology as well as some of its current applications.

Drug Stability

Potential sources for drug instability

Since proteins and nucleic acids are notoriously vulnerable to numerous chemical and physical stressors, stability problems frequently arise in their microencapsulation. The instability problem results in two significant issues:

1) Incomplete and little release of the functional drugs and

2) Immunogenicity or toxicity concern for the degraded or aggregated drugs.

Despite the fact that the primary causes of the instability may change based on the type of medicine, the following factors are frequently cited as potential contributors. The most popular approach for encapsulating most water-soluble medicines, including proteins, peptides, and nucleic acids, is the double-emulsion solvent removal method. Contrarily, it is frequently discovered that these medications are harmed at water/organic solvent (w/o) interfaces. For instance, after centrifuging the emulsion, roughly 40% of the carbonic anhydrase was recovered at the interface when an aqueous solution of carbonic anhydrase was subjected to vortex mixing in the presence of methylene chloride.

Denaturation of the protein medicines can also be brought about by direct contact with the organic solvent. In highly hydrophobic conditions, proteins that are dissolved or suspended in organic solvents encounter, their functional configurations are easily altered. The shear tensions that the emulsion technologies produce are also unfavorable circumstances. The shear rate helps the protein medicines aggregate, especially when it's combined with another adverse circumstance.

Strategies to address the instability issues

The stability of the encapsulated pharmaceuticals has been improved using a variety of strategies. Table 5 highlights alternative strategies based on the causes of inactivation. A novel microencapsulation technique was created recently in an effort to work with most of the above techniques. This novel technique, known as the "solvent exchange approach," relies on interfacial mass transfer between two contacting liquids to produce microcapsules that resemble reservoirs. A technique for creating microcapsules is shown in Fig. 3. Using ink-jet nozzles, a series of droplets from an aqueous drug solution and a polymer solution are independently created, and then they are made to collide in the air. Due to the difference in surface tension and incompatibility of the two liquids, the two liquid phases are split as a core and a membrane within the fused micro droplets after the collision. This approach may provide a number of benefits. First off, the procedure uses a gentle drop generation protocol rather than potentially harmful circumstances like an emulsification stage. Second, only the interface at the surface of the core exhibits unfavorable interactions between protein and organic solvent or polymer matrix in mononuclear microcapsules. According to a recent study, these reservoir-type microcapsules may release the encapsulated lysozyme for more than 50 days with a nearly zero-order kinetics. The functional integrity of the liberated lysozyme indicates that the protein survived microencapsulation without losing biological activity. Third, compared to conventional techniques, there is more freedom in selecting the organic solvent for polymers. Thus, it is possible to minimize worries about the toxicity of leftover solvents, particularly methylene chloride.

Table 5: Common inactivation sources of encapsulated proteins and the stabilization strategies

Inactivation source	**Stabilization strategy**
Exposure to w/o interfaces	Reducing or avoiding denaturation at w/o interfaces by including protective excipients; employing anhydrous microencapsulation processes.
Exposure to the hydrophobic organic solvent	Using more hydrophilic solvents such as Ethyl acetate and methyl ethyl ketone.
Physical stresses during preparation	Reducing physical stresses by eliminating the emulsification step and employing low temperature processes.
Acidification of the microenvironment	Counteracting acidification by co-encapsulating antacid excipients; increasing permeability of the polymer matrix; modifying degradation characteristics of the polymer.
Interaction between protein and polymer	Preventing adsorption by modifying hydrophilicity of the polymer surface; pre-entrapment of protein in the hydrophilic core; Including adsorption competitors.

Control of Drug Release

The rates of polymer degradation, the structural characteristics of the microparticles, and the distribution of the medications inside the particle matrix all affect how quickly biodegradable polymer microparticles release drugs. The creation of conveniently programmable release profiles is the ultimate objective of microparticle systems in controlled drug delivery, and this objective has been approached from a variety of angles.

Size control

The release rate is known to be significantly influenced by particle sizes. Depending on the drug release mechanism, the effects change. Smaller microparticles have a tendency to release drugs at a relatively high rate because of their large surface area and short diffusion distance when the drug release is primarily controlled by diffusion, which is typically the case during the early stage of release from polymeric microparticles or hydrogel-based microparticles. The particle size, on the other hand, regulates the release rate by impacting additional aspects including medication distribution and polymer degradation rate when the release is dependent on polymer degradation.

RECENT APPLICATIONS OF THE MICROPARTICLE SYSTEMS

Microparticle systems can be used for a variety of purposes other than local or sustained distribution. Below, a select few samples are provided. Microparticles constructed of these polymers have been researched as prospective oral drug delivery methods ever since it was discovered that bioerodible hydrophobic polyanhydrides, such as poly (fumaric-co-sebacicanhydride), demonstrated high bioadhesiveness. The hydrogen bonding connections between mucin and carboxylic acid groups that develop during the polymer erosion in this instance are what give rise to the bioadhesiveness. Additionally, the small size of microparticles offers benefits by encouraging formulation uptake by cells. The bioadhesive microparticles have demonstrated improved oral bioavailability of dicumarol, insulin, and DNA by utilizing both the tiny size of microparticles and the chemical characteristics of the polymeric system. In order to deliver DNA vaccines, which allow for prolonged immune responses by persistent release of DNA encoding a protein antigen, polymeric microspheres have been employed. It is well known that macrophages and antigen-presenting cells preferentially absorb 10 mm particles by phagocytosis. In the original research, poly(lactic-co-glycolic acid) was utilized as an encapsulating polymer with encouraging outcomes. The sluggish release rate of PLGA particles, which does not keep up with the life span of the target cells like dendritic cells, and acidification of the microenvironment are drawbacks of using them to deliver DNA vaccines. Recently, pH-triggered biodegradable polymers based on poly (ortho esters) and poly (b- amino esters were used to provide for quick and adjustable release while preventing internal acidification. These DNA-loaded microparticles were successfully absorbed by antigen-presenting cells, which improved immune response and greatly reduced in vivo tumor challenges.

References:

1. Gullapalli RP. Soft gelatin capsules (softgels). J Pharm Sci. 2010 Oct;99(10):4107-48. doi: 10.1002/jps.22151. PMID: 20737624.
2. Gullapalli RP, Mazzitelli CL. Gelatin and Non-Gelatin Capsule Dosage Forms. J Pharm Sci. 2017 Jun;106(6):1453-1465. doi: 10.1016/j.xphs.2017.02.006. Epub 2017 Feb 14. PMID: 28209365.
3. MS Patel, FSS Morton, & H Seager (1989) "Advances in softgel formulation technology" Manuf Chem, July 26–28.
4. LA Augsburger (1995) "Hard and soft gelatin capsules" in Modern Pharmaceutics GS Banker & CT Rhodes, Eds., Marcel Dekker, Inc.: New York, NY, pp 395–440.

FSC
www.fsc.org
MIX
Papier | Fördert gute Waldnutzung
FSC® C083411

Kolibri 360 GmbH
Ferdinand-Jühlke-Straße 7
99095 Erfurt, Deutschland
produktsicherheit@kolibri360.de

Druck:
CPI Druckdienstleistungen GmbH
im Auftrag der
Kolibri 360 GmbH
Ferdinand-Jühlke-Str. 7
99095 Erfurt